DIABETES

203nm

Written by: Nester Kadzviti Murira PhD,M.Med Ed.

This is a record of your health.

Carry this book wherever you go.

The information inside this book could save your life.

<u>Show this book to health personnel.</u>

Name:..

Address...

....

....

....

Tel...

Hospital/Dr...

Dr'sAddress..

....

....

Next **of** **Kin**

....

....

Tel...

My Current Medication is:

1………………………………………………………………

2………………………………………………………………

3………………………………………………………………

4………………………………………………………………

5………………………………………………………………

Allergies………………………………………………………
……………………………………………………………………
……………………………………………………………………
……………………………………………………………………
……………………………………………………………………
……………………………………………………………………

DIABETES

Starches and sugars in the food one eats are used to provide the body with energy. The rest of the starches are kept in the body where they are stored in muscle or converted to fat that provides warmth to the body. The body requires adequate amounts of a hormone called insulin to manage the sugars and starches that one takes in.

- Insulin is produced by the pancreas, an organ that lies below the stomach.
- If the body fails to produce enough amounts of insulin. Large amounts of sugars that the body cannot readily use remain in the blood.
- Some of the sugar leaves the body through the urine but the remaining sugar in the body affects many parts of the body causing one to fall ill and loose consciousness.
- If one's body produces a lot of insulin and there is little sugar in one's blood, the individual falls ill, becomes very weak, faints and falls unconscious.

- Diabetes follows the family tree and affects men and women as well as children.

How can one tell that they have diabetes?

- One feels very hungry frequently even after a good meal and eats large amounts of food to satisfy their hunger.
- One feels unusually thirsty and drinks large amounts of fluids frequently.
- One passes large amounts of urine and wakes up at night frequently to empty the bladder.
- Some people may put on excessive weight, some especially the young, may loose weight.

Other symptoms of diabetes

- One has sweet smelling breath
- One may have attacks of thrush and feels itchy especially on the external genital organs.
- One may have wounds that take long or fail to heal.
- One may have gradually poor eye sight.
- One may experience unexplained fainting attacks.

How can one look after oneself once diagnosed with the condition?

- Keep your appointments with the doctor.
- Expect frequent blood tests to monitor the condition.
- One may be hospitalised as an emergency if the blood sugar levels are unstable.
- It is advisable to always carry a Medic Alert or a booklet that states that one is diabetic in case of emergency.
- If on medication always have something to eat.
- Have glucose sweets on you in case you feel excessively hungry and need to boost energy,
- Control body weight by reducing the intake of starches, sugars and fats in the diet.
- Avoid tight shoes as they can bruise toes and cause wounds
- Report infections to health personnel early.

Blood Tests Results

Date	Test	Results	Medication

Blood Tests Results

Date	Test	Results	Medication

DIABETES IN PREGNANCY

- One may not be aware of the condition until after tests.
- A woman with a family history of diabetes is more likely to have diabetes in pregnancy.
- Women with excessive weight in pregnancy are likely to have diabetes in pregnancy.

How does diabetes affect pregnancy?

- One gains excessive weight
- One carries heavily; the baby is bigger than expected and therefore the individual is likely to have complicated labour that requires an operative delivery.
- The large amounts of sugar in the body affects the baby's breathing and this requires that the baby is delivered early (prematurely) to save the baby.
- Due to the excessive weight complications such as high blood pressure may arise.

How does pregnancy affect diabetes?

- If you already know that you have diabetes on falling pregnant, expect the symptoms of the condition to increase in pregnancy.
- Report pregnancy to health personnel as soon as you know that you are pregnant. You medications is likely to be adjusted.
- Expect more tests in pregnancy
- You must monitor fetal movements
- Expect early delivery of a premature baby by Caesarean Section

Have you eaten?

Have you taken your medication?

Please tick after taking medication.

Date/Day	Morning	Afternoon	Evening	Glucose Test
Monday				
Tuesday				
Wednesday				
Thursday				
Friday				
Saturday				
Sunday				

Have you eaten?

Have you taken your medication?

Please tick after taking medication.

Date/Day	Morning	Afternoon	Evening	Glucose Test
Monday				
Tuesday				
Wednesday				
Thursday				
Friday				
Saturday				
Sunday				

Have you eaten?

Have you taken your medication?

Please tick after taking medication.

Date/Day	Morning	Afternoon	Evening	Glucose Test
Monday				
Tuesday				
Wednesday				
Thursday				
Friday				
Saturday				
Sunday				

Have you eaten?

Have you taken your medication?

Please tick after taking medication.

Date/Day	Morning	Afternoon	Evening	Glucose Test
Monday				
Tuesday				
Wednesday				
Thursday				
Friday				
Saturday				
Sunday				

Have you eaten?

Have you taken your medication?

Please tick after taking medication.

Date/Day	Morning	Afternoon	Evening	Glucose Test
Monday				
Tuesday				
Wednesday				
Thursday				
Friday				
Saturday				
Sunday				

Have you eaten?

Have you taken your medication?

Please tick after taking medication.

Date/Day	Morning	Afternoon	Evening	Glucose Test
Monday				
Tuesday				
Wednesday				
Thursday				
Friday				
Saturday				
Sunday				

Have you eaten?

Have you taken your medication?

Please tick after taking medication.

Date/Day	Morning	Afternoon	Evening	
Monday				
Tuesday				
Wednesday				
Thursday				
Friday				
Saturday				
Sunday				

Have you eaten?

Have you taken your medication?

Tick after taking medication.

Date/Day	Morning	Afternoon	Evening	Glucose Test
Monday				
Tuesday				
Wednesday				
Thursday				
Friday				
Saturday				
Sunday				

Have you eaten?

Have you taken your medication?

Please tick after taking medication.

Date/Day	Morning	Afternoon	Evening	Glucose Test
Monday				
Tuesday				
Wednesday				
Thursday				
Friday				
Saturday				
Sunday				

Have you eaten?

Have you taken your medication?

Please tick after taking medication.

Date/Day	Morning	Afternoon	Evening	Glucose Test
Monday				
Tuesday				
Wednesday				
Thursday				
Friday				
Saturday				
Sunday				

Have you eaten?

Have you taken your medication?

Please tick after taking medication.

Date/Day	Morning	Afternoon	Evening	Glucose Test
Monday				
Tuesday				
Wednesday				
Thursday				
Friday				
Saturday				
Sunday				

Have you eaten?

Have you taken your medication?

Please tick after taking medication.

Date/Day	Morning	Afternoon	Evening	Glucose Test
Monday				
Tuesday				
Wednesday				
Thursday				
Friday				
Saturday				
Sunday